The
Lifestyle Design
Planner

Stacy Fisher

8 Dimensions of Self-Care

Emotive
How you express yourself

Luminescent
How you illuminate your inner truth

Systemic
How you eat, move and rest

Financial
How you allocate your resources

Environmental
How you harmonize with nature

Cognitive
How you think

Relational
How you connect with others

Aptitudinal
How you contribute to the world

LivingUpp

LivingUpp
A Lifestyle Design Company

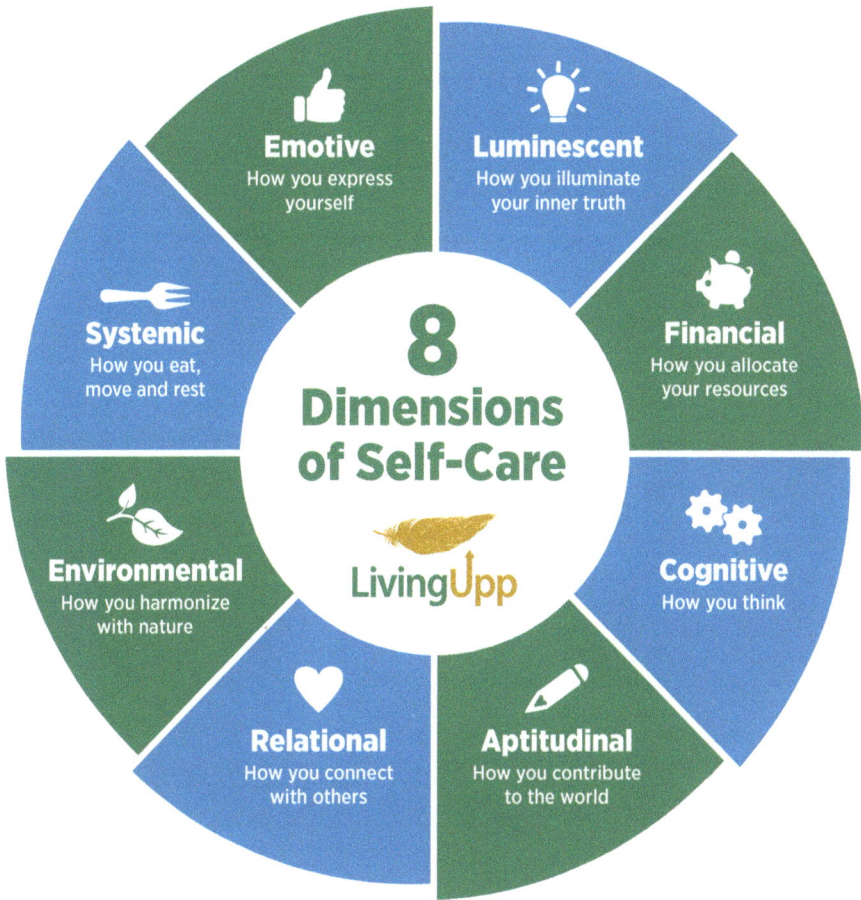

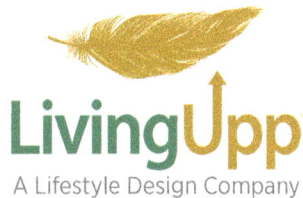

Published by Intrinsic Publishing   ISBN: 978-0-9974853-4-9

Get tips for using this planner at www.LivingUpp.com/Planner.

Contents

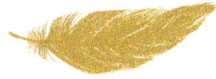

A Note from Stacy...8

The 8 Dimensions of Self-Care.................................10

How to Rate Your 8...11

Self Discovery Worksheet...12

Yearly Calendar..14

Yearly Planning...16

Vision Board...18

Quarterly Planning..20

Monthly Planning..24

Weekly Planning...72

Future Planning..282

Self-Care Activities...292

Bonus...298

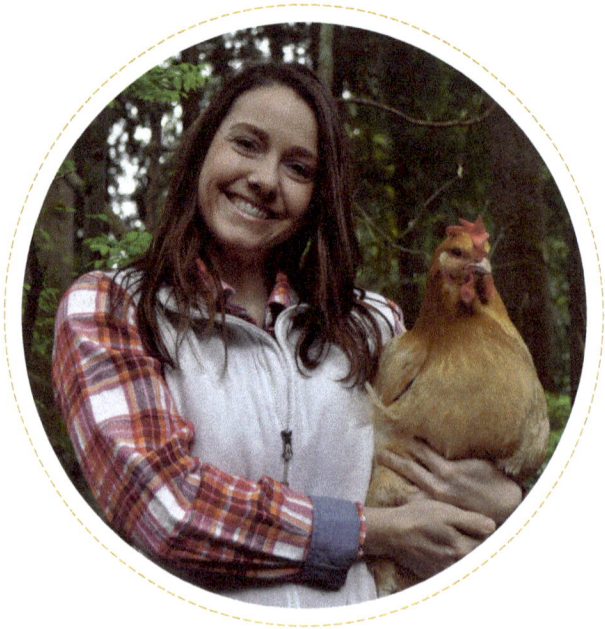

A note from Stacy

If planners and office supplies make you giddy, then you're in good company. The Lifestyle Design Planner will help you create more ease and better health by keeping you focused on what's most important.

For years I've been searching for the perfect planner to keep my hot mess of a life in order — one that provides enough structure to keep me organized without limiting my creativity. But with each new planner came the eventual realization that something was missing. It was either too big, too heavy, too chintzy, or lacked a certain something that led me to continue my search for yet another planner.

I wanted a planner that was pretty yet durable, inspiring but uncluttered, and most of all I wanted a system that would help me organize and simplify my life. I needed a way to take meeting notes, create task lists, track my goals, plan my future, hold myself accountable, and jot down ideas as they came to me. And I wanted it to fit easily into my handbag. (Is that too much to ask?) With these requirements in mind, the Lifestyle Design Planner was born.

Self-care is the central theme of this planner. That's because good health is your greatest asset; it's what helps you continue to be in service to others. Using LivingUpp's 8-dimensional self-care framework, you can easily assess and prioritize the areas of your life that need the most attention so you can invest your time and energy efficiently.

For tips and instructions on how to get the most out of the Lifestyle Design Planner, visit **LivingUpp.com/Planner.** (We didn't want to clutter up your pages with information you may or may not need.)

Cheers to creating more ease and better health!

The 8 dimensions of self-care

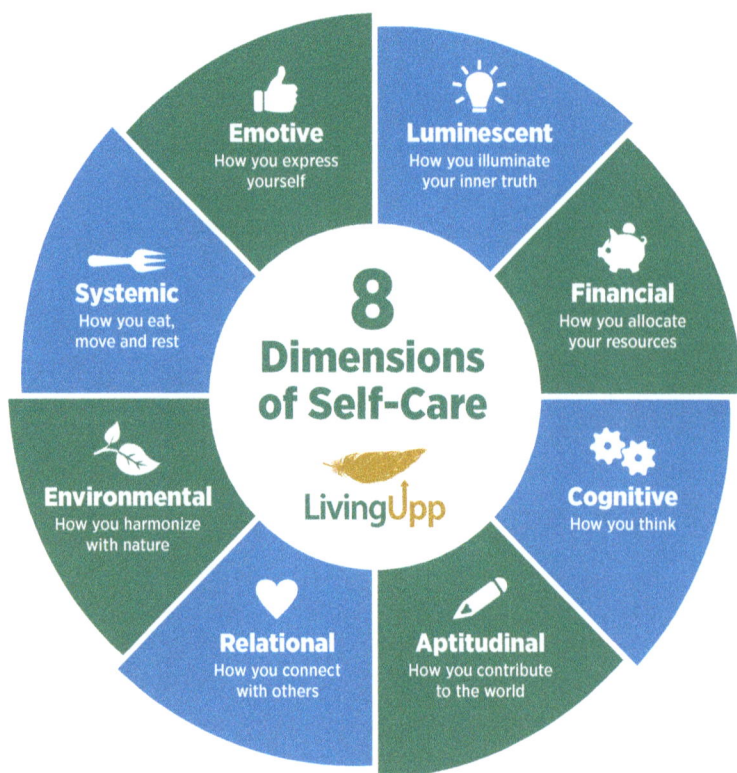

8 Dimensions of Self-Care
LivingUpp

- **Emotive** — How you express yourself
- **Luminescent** — How you illuminate your inner truth
- **Financial** — How you allocate your resources
- **Cognitive** — How you think
- **Aptitudinal** — How you contribute to the world
- **Relational** — How you connect with others
- **Environmental** — How you harmonize with nature
- **Systemic** — How you eat, move and rest

S » SYSTEMIC How you eat, move and rest.

E » EMOTIVE How you express yourself.

L » LUMINESCENT How you illuminate your inner truth.

F » FINANCIAL How you allocate your resources.

C » COGNITIVE How you think.

A » APTITUDINAL How you contribute to the world.

R » RELATIONAL How you connect with others.

E » ENVIRONMENTAL How you harmonize with nature.

How to rate your 8

Using a scale of 1 to 10
(with 10 being the highest),
rank how well you're
supporting yourself in each
dimension right now.
Don't overthink it; go with your gut.

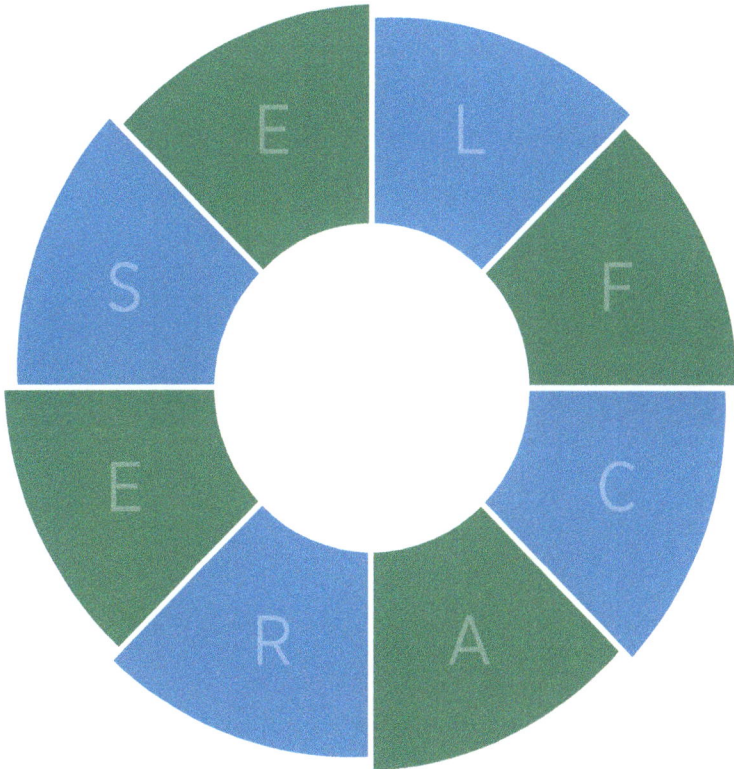

Self-Discovery Worksheet

Systemic: How you eat, move and rest

Currently

1 2 3 4 5 6 7 8 9 10

Future Vision

What would make it a 10 for you?

....

....

....

....

....

Emotive: How you express yourself

Currently

1 2 3 4 5 6 7 8 9 10

Future Vision

What would make it a 10 for you?

....

....

....

....

....

Luminescent: How you illuminate your inner truth

Currently

1 2 3 4 5 6 7 8 9 10

Future Vision

What would make it a 10 for you?

....

....

....

....

....

Financial: How you allocate your resources

Currently

1 2 3 4 5 6 7 8 9 10

Future Vision

What would make it a 10 for you?

....

....

....

....

....

Instructions: In the left column, rate each self-care dimension on a scale of 1 to 10 (with 10 being the highest) as it pertains to your life currently. In the right column, consider what would make this particular dimension a "10" for you, and use the box below to describe what you envision.

Cognitive: How you think

Currently

1 2 3 4 5 6 7 8 9 10

Future Vision

What would make it a 10 for you?

....
....
....
....
....

Aptitudinal: How you contribute to the world

Currently

1 2 3 4 5 6 7 8 9 10

Future Vision

What would make it a 10 for you?

....
....
....
....
....

Relational: How you connect with others

Currently

1 2 3 4 5 6 7 8 9 10

Future Vision

What would make it a 10 for you?

....
....
....
....
....

Environmental: How you harmonize with nature

Currently

1 2 3 4 5 6 7 8 9 10

Future Vision

What would make it a 10 for you?

....
....
....
....
....

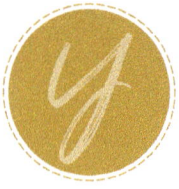

Yearly Calendar

JANUARY

FEBRUARY

MARCH

APRIL

MAY

JUNE

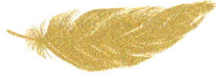

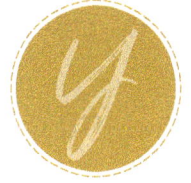

JULY

AUGUST

SEPTEMBER

OCTOBER

NOVEMBER

DECEMBER

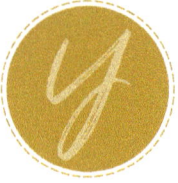

Year............

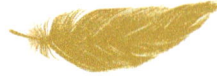

Theme Words

....

....

....

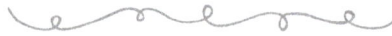

Core Values

....

....

....

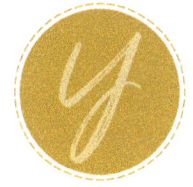

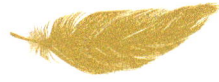

8 Dimensional Plan

Systemic

....

Emotive

....

Luminescent

....

Financial

....

Cognitive

....

Aptitudinal

....

Relational

....

Environmental

....

What do you want
to do, have, be, or feel?

Vision Board

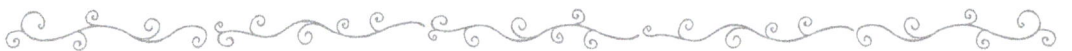

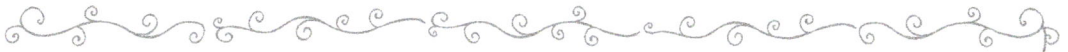

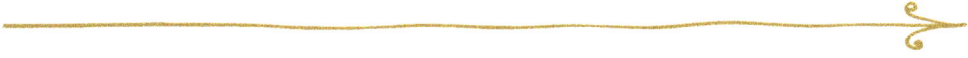

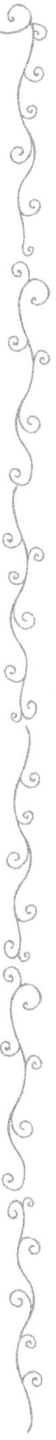

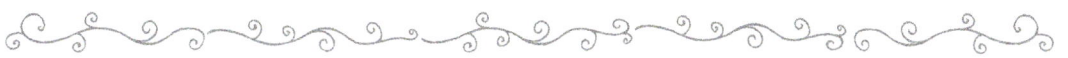

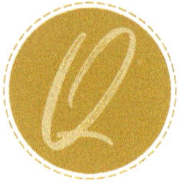

Quarter ....

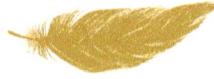

8 Dimensional Plan

Systemic

....

Emotive

....

Luminescent

....

Financial

....

Cognitive

....

Aptitudinal

....

Relational

....

Environmental

....

Quarter ....

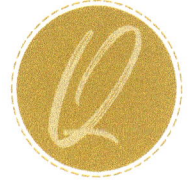

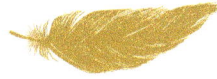

8 Dimensional Plan

Systemic
....

Emotive
....

Luminescent
....

Financial
....

Cognitive
....

Aptitudinal
....

Relational
....

Environmental
....

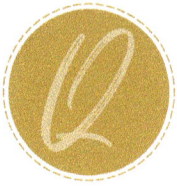

Quarter ....

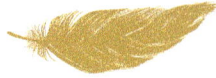

8 Dimensional Plan

Systemic ....

Emotive ....

Luminescent ....

Financial ....

Cognitive ....

Aptitudinal ....

Relational ....

Environmental ....

Quarter ....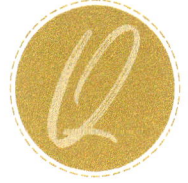

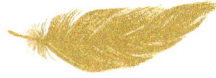

8 Dimensional Plan

Systemic
....

Emotive
....

Luminescent
....

Financial
....

Cognitive
....

Aptitudinal
....

Relational
....

Environmental
....

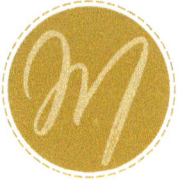

Month ....

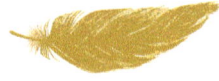

8 Dimensional Plan

Systemic
....

Emotive
....

Luminescent
....

Financial
....

Cognitive
....

Aptitudinal
....

Relational
....

Environmental
....

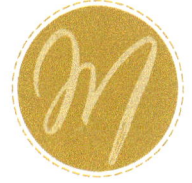

Monthly Tracker

Activity	1	2	3	4	5	6	7	8	9	10	11	12	13	14	15	16
	17	18	19	20	21	22	23	24	25	26	27	28	29	30	31	
Activity	1	2	3	4	5	6	7	8	9	10	11	12	13	14	15	16
	17	18	19	20	21	22	23	24	25	26	27	28	29	30	31	
Activity	1	2	3	4	5	6	7	8	9	10	11	12	13	14	15	16
	17	18	19	20	21	22	23	24	25	26	27	28	29	30	31	
Activity	1	2	3	4	5	6	7	8	9	10	11	12	13	14	15	16
	17	18	19	20	21	22	23	24	25	26	27	28	29	30	31	

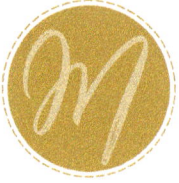

Monthly Calendar

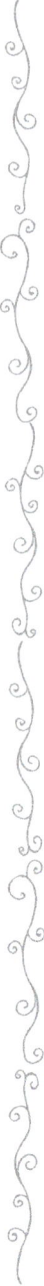

MONDAY	TUESDAY	WEDNESDAY

Month

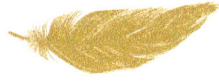

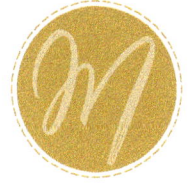

THURSDAY	FRIDAY	SATURDAY	SUNDAY

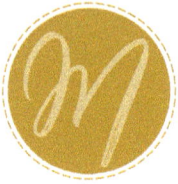

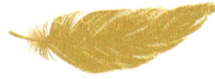

Month ....

8 Dimensional Plan

Systemic ....

Emotive ....

Luminescent ....

Financial ....

Cognitive ....

Aptitudinal ....

Relational ....

Environmental ....

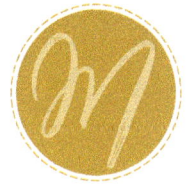

Monthly Tracker

Activity	1	2	3	4	5	6	7	8	9	10	11	12	13	14	15	16
	17	18	19	20	21	22	23	24	25	26	27	28	29	30	31	
Activity	1	2	3	4	5	6	7	8	9	10	11	12	13	14	15	16
	17	18	19	20	21	22	23	24	25	26	27	28	29	30	31	
Activity	1	2	3	4	5	6	7	8	9	10	11	12	13	14	15	16
	17	18	19	20	21	22	23	24	25	26	27	28	29	30	31	
Activity	1	2	3	4	5	6	7	8	9	10	11	12	13	14	15	16
	17	18	19	20	21	22	23	24	25	26	27	28	29	30	31	

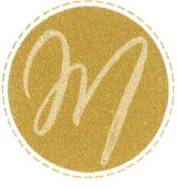

Monthly Calendar

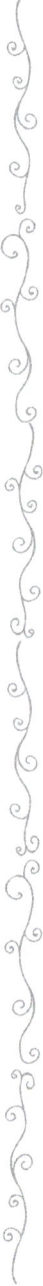

MONDAY	TUESDAY	WEDNESDAY

Month

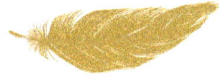

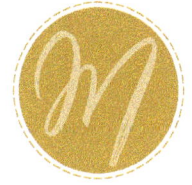

THURSDAY	FRIDAY	SATURDAY	SUNDAY

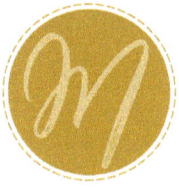

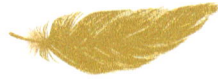

Month ....

8 Dimensional Plan

Systemic ....

Emotive ....

Luminescent ....

Financial ....

Cognitive ....

Aptitudinal ....

Relational ....

Environmental ....

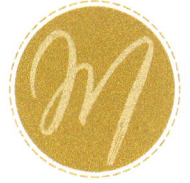

Monthly Tracker

Activity	1	2	3	4	5	6	7	8	9	10	11	12	13	14	15	16
	17	18	19	20	21	22	23	24	25	26	27	28	29	30	31	
Activity	1	2	3	4	5	6	7	8	9	10	11	12	13	14	15	16
	17	18	19	20	21	22	23	24	25	26	27	28	29	30	31	
Activity	1	2	3	4	5	6	7	8	9	10	11	12	13	14	15	16
	17	18	19	20	21	22	23	24	25	26	27	28	29	30	31	
Activity	1	2	3	4	5	6	7	8	9	10	11	12	13	14	15	16
	17	18	19	20	21	22	23	24	25	26	27	28	29	30	31	

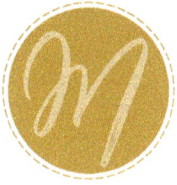

Monthly Calendar

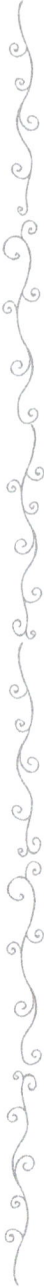

MONDAY	TUESDAY	WEDNESDAY

Month

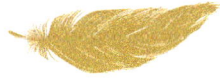

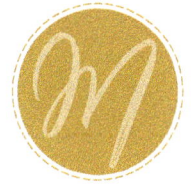

THURSDAY	FRIDAY	SATURDAY	SUNDAY

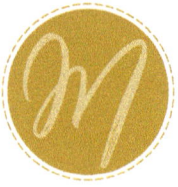

Month ....

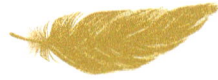

8 Dimensional Plan

Systemic ....

Emotive ....

Luminescent ....

Financial ....

Cognitive ....

Aptitudinal ....

Relational ....

Environmental ....

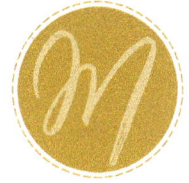

Monthly Tracker

Activity	1	2	3	4	5	6	7	8	9	10	11	12	13	14	15	16
	17	18	19	20	21	22	23	24	25	26	27	28	29	30	31	
Activity	1	2	3	4	5	6	7	8	9	10	11	12	13	14	15	16
	17	18	19	20	21	22	23	24	25	26	27	28	29	30	31	
Activity	1	2	3	4	5	6	7	8	9	10	11	12	13	14	15	16
	17	18	19	20	21	22	23	24	25	26	27	28	29	30	31	
Activity	1	2	3	4	5	6	7	8	9	10	11	12	13	14	15	16
	17	18	19	20	21	22	23	24	25	26	27	28	29	30	31	

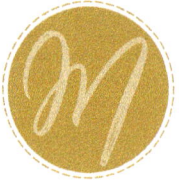

Monthly Calendar

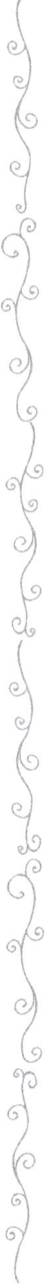

MONDAY	TUESDAY	WEDNESDAY

Month

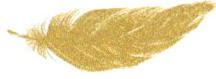

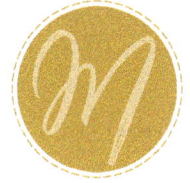

THURSDAY	FRIDAY	SATURDAY	SUNDAY

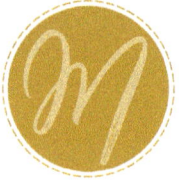

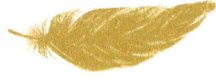 Month ....

8 Dimensional Plan

Systemic ....

Emotive ....

Luminescent ....

Financial ....

Cognitive ....

Aptitudinal ....

Relational ....

Environmental ....

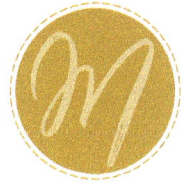

Monthly Tracker

Activity	1	2	3	4	5	6	7	8	9	10	11	12	13	14	15	16
	17	18	19	20	21	22	23	24	25	26	27	28	29	30	31	
Activity	1	2	3	4	5	6	7	8	9	10	11	12	13	14	15	16
	17	18	19	20	21	22	23	24	25	26	27	28	29	30	31	
Activity	1	2	3	4	5	6	7	8	9	10	11	12	13	14	15	16
	17	18	19	20	21	22	23	24	25	26	27	28	29	30	31	
Activity	1	2	3	4	5	6	7	8	9	10	11	12	13	14	15	16
	17	18	19	20	21	22	23	24	25	26	27	28	29	30	31	

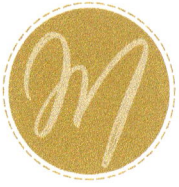

Monthly Calendar

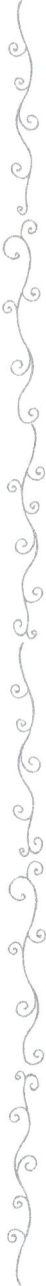

MONDAY	TUESDAY	WEDNESDAY

Month

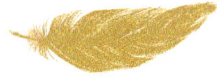

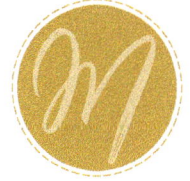

THURSDAY	FRIDAY	SATURDAY	SUNDAY

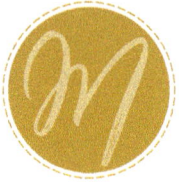

Month ....

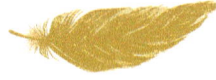

8 Dimensional Plan

Systemic ....

Emotive ....

Luminescent ....

Financial ....

Cognitive ....

Aptitudinal ....

Relational ....

Environmental ....

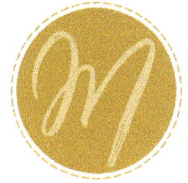

Monthly Tracker

Activity	1	2	3	4	5	6	7	8	9	10	11	12	13	14	15	16
	17	18	19	20	21	22	23	24	25	26	27	28	29	30	31	
Activity	1	2	3	4	5	6	7	8	9	10	11	12	13	14	15	16
	17	18	19	20	21	22	23	24	25	26	27	28	29	30	31	
Activity	1	2	3	4	5	6	7	8	9	10	11	12	13	14	15	16
	17	18	19	20	21	22	23	24	25	26	27	28	29	30	31	
Activity	1	2	3	4	5	6	7	8	9	10	11	12	13	14	15	16
	17	18	19	20	21	22	23	24	25	26	27	28	29	30	31	

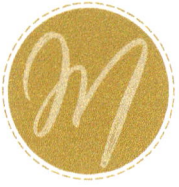

Monthly Calendar

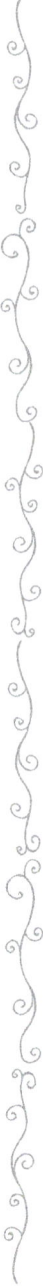

MONDAY	TUESDAY	WEDNESDAY

Month

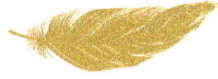

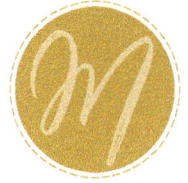

THURSDAY	FRIDAY	SATURDAY	SUNDAY

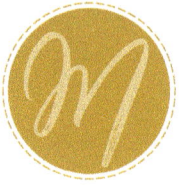

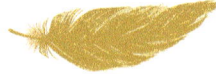

8 Dimensional Plan

Systemic ....

Emotive ....

Luminescent ....

Financial ....

Cognitive ....

Aptitudinal ....

Relational ....

Environmental ....

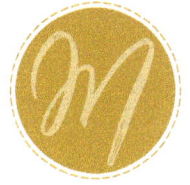

Monthly Tracker

Activity	1	2	3	4	5	6	7	8	9	10	11	12	13	14	15	16
	17	18	19	20	21	22	23	24	25	26	27	28	29	30	31	
Activity	1	2	3	4	5	6	7	8	9	10	11	12	13	14	15	16
	17	18	19	20	21	22	23	24	25	26	27	28	29	30	31	
Activity	1	2	3	4	5	6	7	8	9	10	11	12	13	14	15	16
	17	18	19	20	21	22	23	24	25	26	27	28	29	30	31	
Activity	1	2	3	4	5	6	7	8	9	10	11	12	13	14	15	16
	17	18	19	20	21	22	23	24	25	26	27	28	29	30	31	

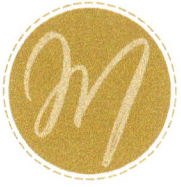

Monthly Calendar

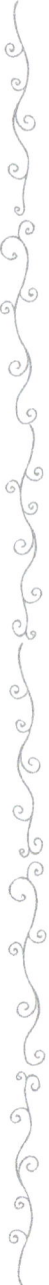

MONDAY	TUESDAY	WEDNESDAY

Month

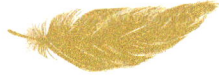

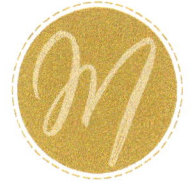

THURSDAY	FRIDAY	SATURDAY	SUNDAY

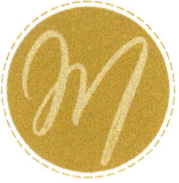

Month ....

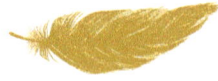

8 Dimensional Plan

Systemic
....

Emotive
....

Luminescent
....

Financial
....

Cognitive
....

Aptitudinal
....

Relational
....

Environmental
....

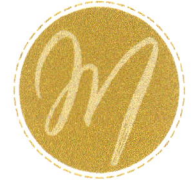

Monthly Tracker

Activity	1	2	3	4	5	6	7	8	9	10	11	12	13	14	15	16
	17	18	19	20	21	22	23	24	25	26	27	28	29	30	31	
Activity	1	2	3	4	5	6	7	8	9	10	11	12	13	14	15	16
	17	18	19	20	21	22	23	24	25	26	27	28	29	30	31	
Activity	1	2	3	4	5	6	7	8	9	10	11	12	13	14	15	16
	17	18	19	20	21	22	23	24	25	26	27	28	29	30	31	
Activity	1	2	3	4	5	6	7	8	9	10	11	12	13	14	15	16
	17	18	19	20	21	22	23	24	25	26	27	28	29	30	31	

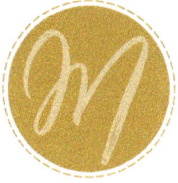

Monthly Calendar

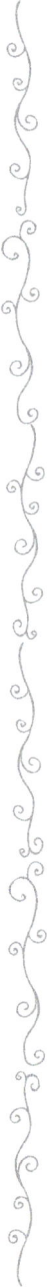

MONDAY	TUESDAY	WEDNESDAY

Month

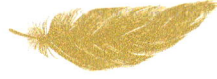

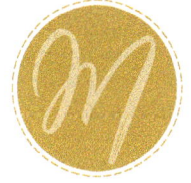

THURSDAY	FRIDAY	SATURDAY	SUNDAY

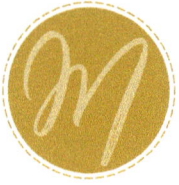

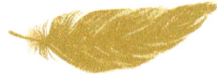

8 Dimensional Plan

Systemic ....

Emotive ....

Luminescent ....

Financial ....

Cognitive ....

Aptitudinal ....

Relational ....

Environmental ....

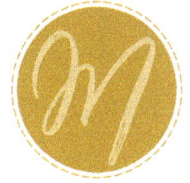

Monthly Tracker

Activity	1	2	3	4	5	6	7	8	9	10	11	12	13	14	15	16
	17	18	19	20	21	22	23	24	25	26	27	28	29	30	31	
Activity	1	2	3	4	5	6	7	8	9	10	11	12	13	14	15	16
	17	18	19	20	21	22	23	24	25	26	27	28	29	30	31	
Activity	1	2	3	4	5	6	7	8	9	10	11	12	13	14	15	16
	17	18	19	20	21	22	23	24	25	26	27	28	29	30	31	
Activity	1	2	3	4	5	6	7	8	9	10	11	12	13	14	15	16
	17	18	19	20	21	22	23	24	25	26	27	28	29	30	31	

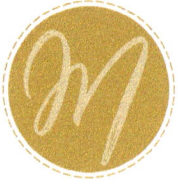

Monthly Calendar

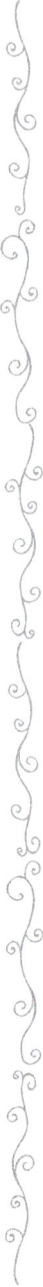

MONDAY	TUESDAY	WEDNESDAY

Month

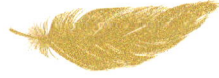

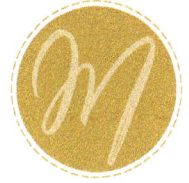

THURSDAY	FRIDAY	SATURDAY	SUNDAY

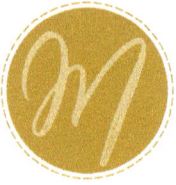

Month ....

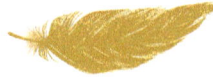

8 Dimensional Plan

Systemic ....

Emotive ....

Luminescent ....

Financial ....

Cognitive ....

Aptitudinal ....

Relational ....

Environmental ....

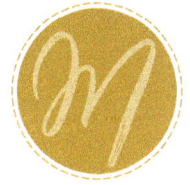

Monthly Tracker

Activity	1	2	3	4	5	6	7	8	9	10	11	12	13	14	15	16
	17	18	19	20	21	22	23	24	25	26	27	28	29	30	31	
Activity	1	2	3	4	5	6	7	8	9	10	11	12	13	14	15	16
	17	18	19	20	21	22	23	24	25	26	27	28	29	30	31	
Activity	1	2	3	4	5	6	7	8	9	10	11	12	13	14	15	16
	17	18	19	20	21	22	23	24	25	26	27	28	29	30	31	
Activity	1	2	3	4	5	6	7	8	9	10	11	12	13	14	15	16
	17	18	19	20	21	22	23	24	25	26	27	28	29	30	31	

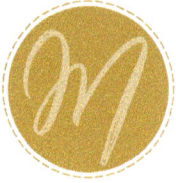

Monthly Calendar

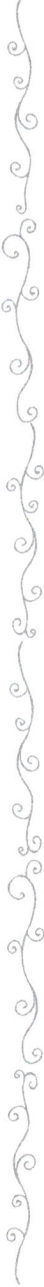

MONDAY	TUESDAY	WEDNESDAY

Month

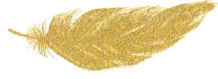

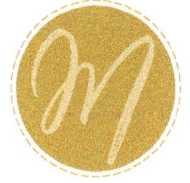

THURSDAY	FRIDAY	SATURDAY	SUNDAY

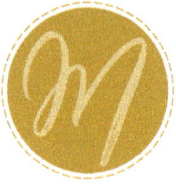

Month ....

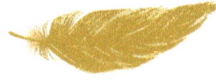

8 Dimensional Plan

Systemic ....

Emotive ....

Luminescent ....

Financial ....

Cognitive ....

Aptitudinal ....

Relational ....

Environmental ....

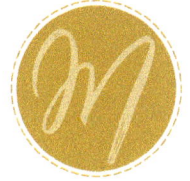

Monthly Tracker

Activity	1	2	3	4	5	6	7	8	9	10	11	12	13	14	15	16
	17	18	19	20	21	22	23	24	25	26	27	28	29	30	31	
Activity	1	2	3	4	5	6	7	8	9	10	11	12	13	14	15	16
	17	18	19	20	21	22	23	24	25	26	27	28	29	30	31	
Activity	1	2	3	4	5	6	7	8	9	10	11	12	13	14	15	16
	17	18	19	20	21	22	23	24	25	26	27	28	29	30	31	
Activity	1	2	3	4	5	6	7	8	9	10	11	12	13	14	15	16
	17	18	19	20	21	22	23	24	25	26	27	28	29	30	31	

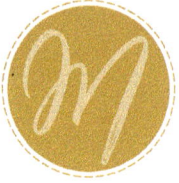

Monthly Calendar

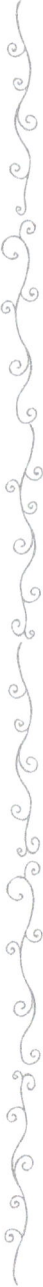

MONDAY	TUESDAY	WEDNESDAY

Month

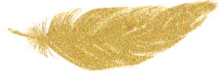

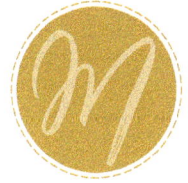

THURSDAY	FRIDAY	SATURDAY	SUNDAY

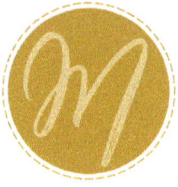

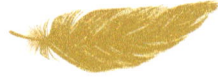

8 Dimensional Plan

Systemic ....

Emotive ....

Luminescent ....

Financial ....

Cognitive ....

Aptitudinal ....

Relational ....

Environmental ....

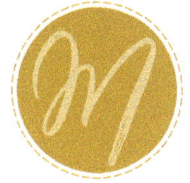

Monthly Tracker

Activity	1	2	3	4	5	6	7	8	9	10	11	12	13	14	15	16
	17	18	19	20	21	22	23	24	25	26	27	28	29	30	31	
Activity	1	2	3	4	5	6	7	8	9	10	11	12	13	14	15	16
	17	18	19	20	21	22	23	24	25	26	27	28	29	30	31	
Activity	1	2	3	4	5	6	7	8	9	10	11	12	13	14	15	16
	17	18	19	20	21	22	23	24	25	26	27	28	29	30	31	
Activity	1	2	3	4	5	6	7	8	9	10	11	12	13	14	15	16
	17	18	19	20	21	22	23	24	25	26	27	28	29	30	31	

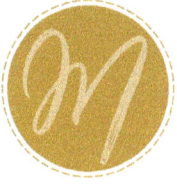

Monthly Calendar

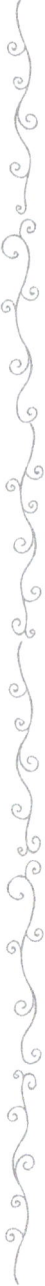

MONDAY	TUESDAY	WEDNESDAY

Month

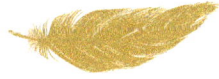

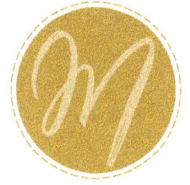

THURSDAY	FRIDAY	SATURDAY	SUNDAY

Weekly

M		T		W	
8		8		8	
9		9		9	
10		10		10	
11		11		11	
12		12		12	
1		1		1	
2		2		2	
3		3		3	
4		4		4	
5		5		5	

T		F		S	
8		8			
9		9			
10		10			
11		11			
12		12			
1		1		S	
2		2			
3		3			
4		4			
5		5			

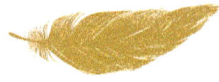

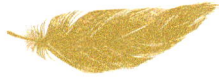

Weekly

M		T		W	
8		8		8	
9		9		9	
10		10		10	
11		11		11	
12		12		12	
1		1		1	
2		2		2	
3		3		3	
4		4		4	
5		5		5	

T		F		S	
8		8			
9		9			
10		10			
11		11			
12		12			
1		1		S	
2		2			
3		3			
4		4			
5		5			

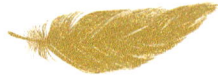

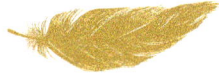

Weekly

M	T	W
8	8	8
9	9	9
10	10	10
11	11	11
12	12	12
1	1	1
2	2	2
3	3	3
4	4	4
5	5	5

-
-
-
-
-

Month ....

T		F		S	
8		8			
9		9			
10		10			
11		11			
12		12			
1		1		S	
2		2			
3		3			
4		4			
5		5			

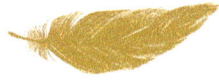

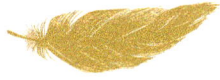

Weekly

M		T		W	
8		8		8	
9		9		9	
10		10		10	
11		11		11	
12		12		12	
1		1		1	
2		2		2	
3		3		3	
4		4		4	
5		5		5	

T		F		S	

8	8
9	9
10	10
11	11
12	12
1	1
2	2
3	3
4	4
5	5

S	

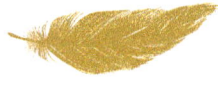

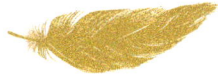

M		T		W	
8		8		8	
9		9		9	
10		10		10	
11		11		11	
12		12		12	
1		1		1	
2		2		2	
3		3		3	
4		4		4	
5		5		5	

Month ....

T		F		S	
8		8			
9		9			
10		10			
11		11			
12		12			
1		1		S	
2		2			
3		3			
4		4			
5		5			

89

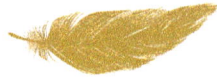

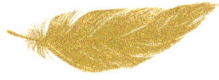

Weekly

M		T		W	
8		8		8	
9		9		9	
10		10		10	
11		11		11	
12		12		12	
1		1		1	
2		2		2	
3		3		3	
4		4		4	
5		5		5	

Month ....

T		F		S	
8		8			
9		9			
10		10			
11		11			
12		12			
1		1		S	
2		2			
3		3			
4		4			
5		5			

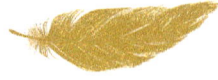

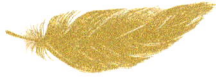

Weekly

M		T		W	
8		8		8	
9		9		9	
10		10		10	
11		11		11	
12		12		12	
1		1		1	
2		2		2	
3		3		3	
4		4		4	
5		5		5	

-
-
-
-
-

Month ....

T		F		S	
8		8			
9		9			
10		10			
11		11			
12		12			
1		1		S	
2		2			
3		3			
4		4			
5		5			

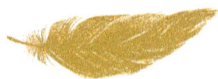

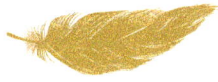

Weekly

M		T		W	

M	T	W
8	8	8
9	9	9
10	10	10
11	11	11
12	12	12
1	1	1
2	2	2
3	3	3
4	4	4
5	5	5

-
-
-
-
-

Month ....

T		F		S	
8		8			
9		9			
10		10			
11		11			
12		12			
1		1		S	
2		2			
3		3			
4		4			
5		5			

SELF CARE SELF CARE SELF CARE SELF CARE

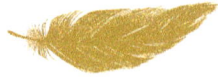

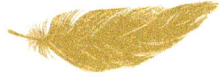

M	T	W
8	8	8
9	9	9
10	10	10
11	11	11
12	12	12
1	1	1
2	2	2
3	3	3
4	4	4
5	5	5

Month

T		F		S	
8		8			
9		9			
10		10			
11		11			
12		12			
1		1		S	
2		2			
3		3			
4		4			
5		5			

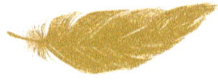

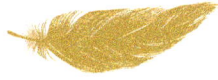

Weekly

M		T		W	
8		8		8	
9		9		9	
10		10		10	
11		11		11	
12		12		12	
1		1		1	
2		2		2	
3		3		3	
4		4		4	
5		5		5	

Month ....

T		F		S	
8		8			
9		9			
10		10			
11		11			
12		12			
1		1		S	
2		2			
3		3			
4		4			
5		5			

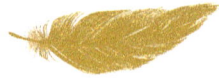

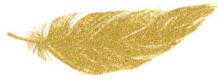

Weekly

M		T		W	
8		8		8	
9		9		9	
10		10		10	
11		11		11	
12		12		12	
1		1		1	
2		2		2	
3		3		3	
4		4		4	
5		5		5	

T		F		S	
8		8			
9		9			
10		10			
11		11			
12		12			
1		1		S	
2		2			
3		3			
4		4			
5		5			

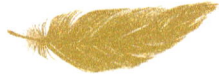

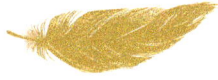

Weekly

M		T		W	
8		8		8	
9		9		9	
10		10		10	
11		11		11	
12		12		12	
1		1		1	
2		2		2	
3		3		3	
4		4		4	
5		5		5	

Month ....

W

T	F	S
8	8	
9	9	
10	10	
11	11	
12	12	S
1	1	
2	2	
3	3	
4	4	
5	5	

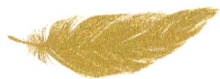

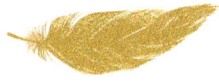

Weekly

M		T		W	
8		8		8	
9		9		9	
10		10		10	
11		11		11	
12		12		12	
1		1		1	
2		2		2	
3		3		3	
4		4		4	
5		5		5	

Month ....

T		F		S	
8		8			
9		9			
10		10			
11		11			
12		12			
1		1		S	
2		2			
3		3			
4		4			
5		5			

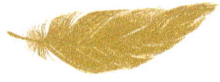

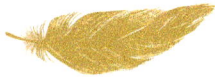

Weekly

	M			T			W	
8			8			8		
9			9			9		
10			10			10		
11			11			11		
12			12			12		
1			1			1		
2			2			2		
3			3			3		
4			4			4		
5			5			5		

Month ....

T		F	
8		8	
9		9	
10		10	
11		11	
12		12	
1		1	
2		2	
3		3	
4		4	
5		5	

S

S

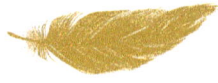

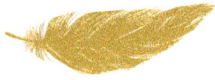

Weekly

M		T		W	
8		8		8	
9		9		9	
10		10		10	
11		11		11	
12		12		12	
1		1		1	
2		2		2	
3		3		3	
4		4		4	
5		5		5	

Month ....

T		F		S	
8		8			
9		9			
10		10			
11		11			
12		12			
1		1		S	
2		2			
3		3			
4		4			
5		5			

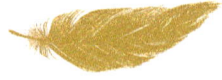

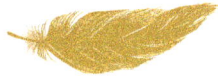

Weekly

M		T		W	
8		8		8	
9		9		9	
10		10		10	
11		11		11	
12		12		12	
1		1		1	
2		2		2	
3		3		3	
4		4		4	
5		5		5	

Month ....

T		F		S	
8		8			
9		9			
10		10			
11		11			
12		12			
1		1		S	
2		2			
3		3			
4		4			
5		5			

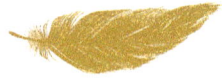

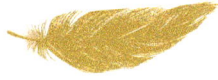

Weekly

M		T		W	
8		8		8	
9		9		9	
10		10		10	
11		11		11	
12		12		12	
1		1		1	
2		2		2	
3		3		3	
4		4		4	
5		5		5	

-
-
-
-
-

Month ....

T		F		S	
8		8			
9		9			
10		10			
11		11			
12		12			
1		1		S	
2		2			
3		3			
4		4			
5		5			

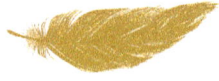

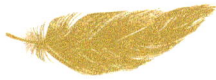

Weekly

	M		T		W	
	8		8		8	
	9		9		9	
	10		10		10	
	11		11		11	
	12		12		12	
	1		1		1	
	2		2		2	
	3		3		3	
	4		4		4	
	5		5		5	

Month ....

T		F		S	
8		8			
9		9			
10		10			
11		11			
12		12			
1		1		S	
2		2			
3		3			
4		4			
5		5			

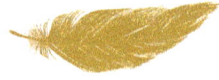

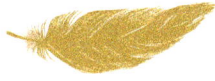

Weekly

M		T		W	
8		8		8	
9		9		9	
10		10		10	
11		11		11	
12		12		12	
1		1		1	
2		2		2	
3		3		3	
4		4		4	
5		5		5	

Month ....

T		F		S	
8		8			
9		9			
10		10			
11		11			
12		12			
1		1		S	
2		2			
3		3			
4		4			
5		5			

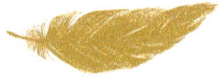

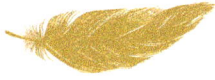

Weekly

M		T		W	
8		8		8	
9		9		9	
10		10		10	
11		11		11	
12		12		12	
1		1		1	
2		2		2	
3		3		3	
4		4		4	
5		5		5	

Month ....

T		F		S	
8		8			
9		9			
10		10			
11		11			
12		12			
1		1		S	
2		2			
3		3			
4		4			
5		5			

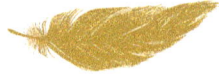

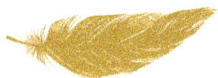

M		T		W	
8		8		8	
9		9		9	
10		10		10	
11		11		11	
12		12		12	
1		1		1	
2		2		2	
3		3		3	
4		4		4	
5		5		5	

Month ....

T		F		S	
8		8			
9		9			
10		10			
11		11			
12		12			
1		1		S	
2		2			
3		3			
4		4			
5		5			

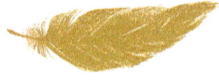

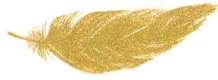

Weekly

M		T		W	
8		8		8	
9		9		9	
10		10		10	
11		11		11	
12		12		12	
1		1		1	
2		2		2	
3		3		3	
4		4		4	
5		5		5	

Month ....

W

T		F		S	
8		8			
9		9			
10		10			
11		11			
12		12			
1		1		**S**	
2		2			
3		3			
4		4			
5		5			

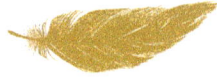

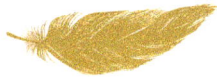

Weekly

	M		T		W	
	8		8		8	
	9		9		9	
	10		10		10	
	11		11		11	
	12		12		12	
	1		1		1	
	2		2		2	
	3		3		3	
	4		4		4	
	5		5		5	

Month ....

T		F		S	
8		8			
9		9			
10		10			
11		11			
12		12			
1		1		S	
2		2			
3		3			
4		4			
5		5			

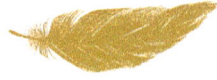

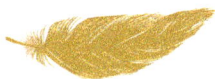

Weekly

M		T		W	
8		8		8	
9		9		9	
10		10		10	
11		11		11	
12		12		12	
1		1		1	
2		2		2	
3		3		3	
4		4		4	
5		5		5	

T		F		S	
8		8			
9		9			
10		10			
11		11			
12		12			
1		1		S	
2		2			
3		3			
4		4			
5		5			

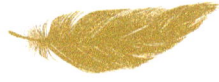

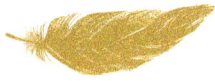

Weekly

M		T		W	
8		8		8	
9		9		9	
10		10		10	
11		11		11	
12		12		12	
1		1		1	
2		2		2	
3		3		3	
4		4		4	
5		5		5	

Month ....

T		F		S	
8		8			
9		9			
10		10			
11		11			
12		12			
1		1		S	
2		2			
3		3			
4		4			
5		5			

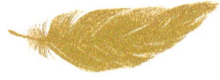

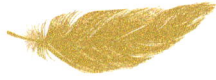

Weekly

M		T		W	
8		8		8	
9		9		9	
10		10		10	
11		11		11	
12		12		12	
1		1		1	
2		2		2	
3		3		3	
4		4		4	
5		5		5	

-
-
-
-
-

Month

T	F	S
8	8	
9	9	
10	10	
11	11	
12	12	
1	1	S
2	2	
3	3	
4	4	
5	5	

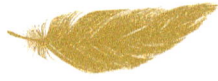

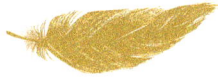

Mid-Year Review

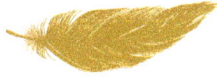

Weekly

	M			T			W	
8			8			8		
9			9			9		
10			10			10		
11			11			11		
12			12			12		
1			1			1		
2			2			2		
3			3			3		
4			4			4		
5			5			5		

Month

T	F	S
8	8	
9	9	
10	10	
11	11	
12	12	
1	1	S
2	2	
3	3	
4	4	
5	5	

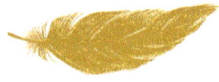

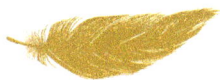

Weekly

M		T		W	
8		8		8	
9		9		9	
10		10		10	
11		11		11	
12		12		12	
1		1		1	
2		2		2	
3		3		3	
4		4		4	
5		5		5	

Month ....

T		F		S	
8		8			
9		9			
10		10			
11		11			
12		12			
1		1		S	
2		2			
3		3			
4		4			
5		5			

183

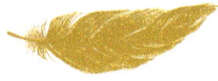

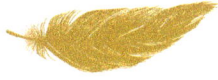

Weekly

	M			T			W	
	8			8			8	
	9			9			9	
	10			10			10	
	11			11			11	
	12			12			12	
	1			1			1	
	2			2			2	
	3			3			3	
	4			4			4	
	5			5			5	

Month ....

T		F		S	
8		8			
9		9			
10		10			
11		11			
12		12			
1		1		S	
2		2			
3		3			
4		4			
5		5			

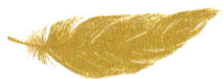

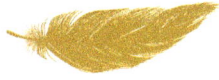

Weekly

M		T		W	
8		8		8	
9		9		9	
10		10		10	
11		11		11	
12		12		12	
1		1		1	
2		2		2	
3		3		3	
4		4		4	
5		5		5	

Month ....

	T		F		S
8		8			
9		9			
10		10			
11		11			
12		12			
1		1		S	
2		2			
3		3			
4		4			
5		5			

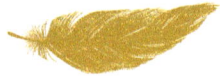

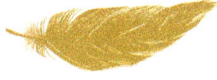

Weekly

M		T		W	
8		8		8	
9		9		9	
10		10		10	
11		11		11	
12		12		12	
1		1		1	
2		2		2	
3		3		3	
4		4		4	
5		5		5	

Month ....

W

T	F	S
8	8	
9	9	
10	10	
11	11	
12	12	
1	1	S
2	2	
3	3	
4	4	
5	5	

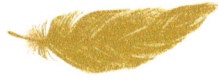

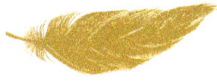

Weekly

M		T		W	
8		8		8	
9		9		9	
10		10		10	
11		11		11	
12		12		12	
1		1		1	
2		2		2	
3		3		3	
4		4		4	
5		5		5	

Month ....

T		F		S	
8		8			
9		9			
10		10			
11		11			
12		12			
1		1		S	
2		2			
3		3			
4		4			
5		5			

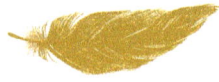

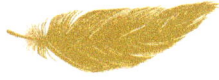

Weekly

M		T		W	
8		8		8	
9		9		9	
10		10		10	
11		11		11	
12		12		12	
1		1		1	
2		2		2	
3		3		3	
4		4		4	
5		5		5	

T	F	S

8	8
9	9
10	10
11	11
12	12
1	1
2	2
3	3
4	4
5	5

S

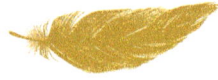

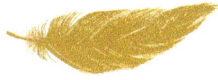

Weekly

M		T		W	
8		8		8	
9		9		9	
10		10		10	
11		11		11	
12		12		12	
1		1		1	
2		2		2	
3		3		3	
4		4		4	
5		5		5	

Month ....

T		F		S	
8		8			
9		9			
10		10			
11		11			
12		12			
1		1		**S**	
2		2			
3		3			
4		4			
5		5			

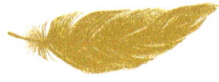

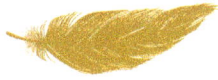

Weekly

	M			T			W	
	8			8			8	
	9			9			9	
	10			10			10	
	11			11			11	
	12			12			12	
	1			1			1	
	2			2			2	
	3			3			3	
	4			4			4	
	5			5			5	

T	F	S
8	8	
9	9	
10	10	
11	11	
12	12	
1	1	S
2	2	
3	3	
4	4	
5	5	

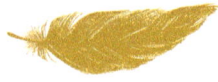

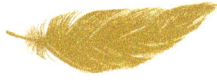

Weekly

M		T		W	
8		8		8	
9		9		9	
10		10		10	
11		11		11	
12		12		12	
1		1		1	
2		2		2	
3		3		3	
4		4		4	
5		5		5	

Month ....

W

T		F		S	
8		8			
9		9			
10		10			
11		11			
12		12			
1		1		S	
2		2			
3		3			
4		4			
5		5			

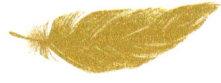

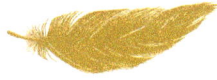

Weekly

M		T		W	
8		8		8	
9		9		9	
10		10		10	
11		11		11	
12		12		12	
1		1		1	
2		2		2	
3		3		3	
4		4		4	
5		5		5	

T		F		S	

8	8
9	9
10	10
11	11
12	12
1	1
2	2
3	3
4	4
5	5

S	

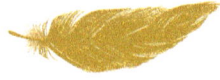

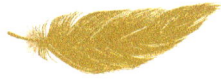

Weekly

M		T		W	
8		8		8	
9		9		9	
10		10		10	
11		11		11	
12		12		12	
1		1		1	
2		2		2	
3		3		3	
4		4		4	
5		5		5	

Month ....

T		F		S	
8		8			
9		9			
10		10			
11		11			
12		12			
1		1		S	
2		2			
3		3			
4		4			
5		5			

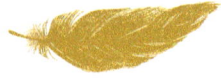

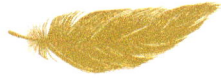

	M			T			W	

-
-
-
-
-

8			8			8		
9			9			9		
10			10			10		
11			11			11		
12			12			12		
1			1			1		
2			2			2		
3			3			3		
4			4			4		
5			5			5		

Month ....

T		F		S	
8		8			
9		9			
10		10			
11		11			
12		12			
1		1		S	
2		2			
3		3			
4		4			
5		5			

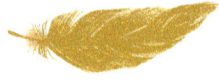

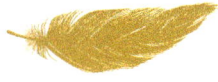

Weekly

M		T		W	
8		8		8	
9		9		9	
10		10		10	
11		11		11	
12		12		12	
1		1		1	
2		2		2	
3		3		3	
4		4		4	
5		5		5	

Month ....

T		F		S	
8		8			
9		9			
10		10			
11		11			
12		12			
1		1		S	
2		2			
3		3			
4		4			
5		5			

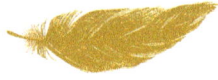

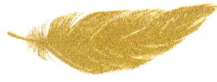

Weekly

M		T		W	
8		8		8	
9		9		9	
10		10		10	
11		11		11	
12		12		12	
1		1		1	
2		2		2	
3		3		3	
4		4		4	
5		5		5	

Month ....

W

T		F		S	
8		8			
9		9			
10		10			
11		11			
12		12			
1		1		S	
2		2			
3		3			
4		4			
5		5			

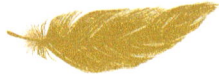

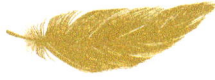

Weekly

M		T		W	
8		8		8	
9		9		9	
10		10		10	
11		11		11	
12		12		12	
1		1		1	
2		2		2	
3		3		3	
4		4		4	
5		5		5	

Month ....

T		F		S	
8		8			
9		9			
10		10			
11		11			
12		12			
1		1		S	
2		2			
3		3			
4		4			
5		5			

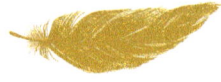

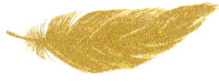

Weekly

M		T		W	
8		8		8	
9		9		9	
10		10		10	
11		11		11	
12		12		12	
1		1		1	
2		2		2	
3		3		3	
4		4		4	
5		5		5	

Month ....

W

T		F		S	
8		8			
9		9			
10		10			
11		11			
12		12			
1		1		S	
2		2			
3		3			
4		4			
5		5			

243

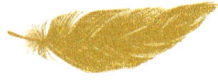

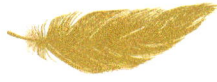

Weekly

M		T		W	
8		8		8	
9		9		9	
10		10		10	
11		11		11	
12		12		12	
1		1		1	
2		2		2	
3		3		3	
4		4		4	
5		5		5	

Month

T	F	S
8	8	
9	9	
10	10	
11	11	
12	12	
1	1	S
2	2	
3	3	
4	4	
5	5	

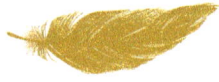

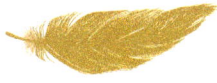

Weekly

M		T		W	
8		8		8	
9		9		9	
10		10		10	
11		11		11	
12		12		12	
1		1		1	
2		2		2	
3		3		3	
4		4		4	
5		5		5	

Month ....

W

T	F	S
8	8	
9	9	
10	10	
11	11	
12	12	
1	1	S
2	2	
3	3	
4	4	
5	5	

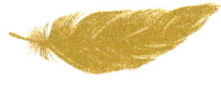

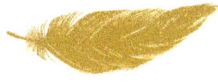

Weekly

M		T		W	
8		8		8	
9		9		9	
10		10		10	
11		11		11	
12		12		12	
1		1		1	
2		2		2	
3		3		3	
4		4		4	
5		5		5	

W

T		F		S	

8	8
9	9
10	10
11	11
12	12
1	1
2	2
3	3
4	4
5	5

S

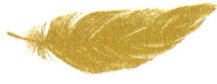

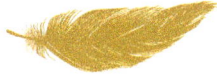

Weekly

M		T		W	
8		8		8	
9		9		9	
10		10		10	
11		11		11	
12		12		12	
1		1		1	
2		2		2	
3		3		3	
4		4		4	
5		5		5	

W

T	F	S

8	8
9	9
10	10
11	11
12	12
1	1
2	2
3	3
4	4
5	5

S

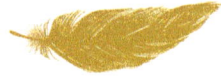

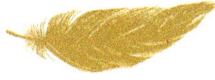

Weekly

M		T		W	
8		8		8	
9		9		9	
10		10		10	
11		11		11	
12		12		12	
1		1		1	
2		2		2	
3		3		3	
4		4		4	
5		5		5	

-
-
-
-
-

Month ....

T		F		S	

8		8	
9		9	
10		10	
11		11	
12		12	
1		1	
2		2	
3		3	
4		4	
5		5	

S

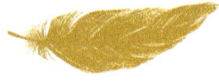

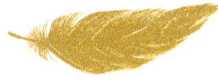

Weekly

	M			T			W	
	8			8			8	
	9			9			9	
	10			10			10	
	11			11			11	
	12			12			12	
	1			1			1	
	2			2			2	
	3			3			3	
	4			4			4	
	5			5			5	

Month _____

T	F	S
8	8	
9	9	
10	10	
11	11	
12	12	
1	1	S
2	2	
3	3	
4	4	
5	5	

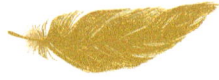

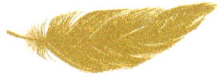

Weekly

M		T		W	
8		8		8	
9		9		9	
10		10		10	
11		11		11	
12		12		12	
1		1		1	
2		2		2	
3		3		3	
4		4		4	
5		5		5	

Month

T	F	S
8	8	
9	9	
10	10	
11	11	
12	12	
1	1	S
2	2	
3	3	
4	4	
5	5	

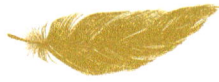

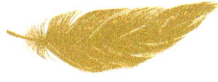

Weekly

M		T		W	
8		8		8	
9		9		9	
10		10		10	
11		11		11	
12		12		12	
1		1		1	
2		2		2	
3		3		3	
4		4		4	
5		5		5	

Month

T		F		S	
8		8			
9		9			
10		10			
11		11			
12		12			
1		1		S	
2		2			
3		3			
4		4			
5		5			

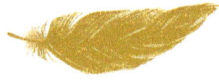

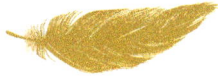

M		T		W	
8		8		8	
9		9		9	
10		10		10	
11		11		11	
12		12		12	
1		1		1	
2		2		2	
3		3		3	
4		4		4	
5		5		5	

Month ....

T		F		S	
8		8			
9		9			
10		10			
11		11			
12		12			
1		1		S	
2		2			
3		3			
4		4			
5		5			

279

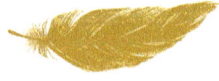

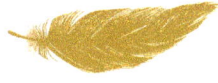

Future Planning

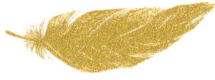

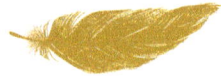

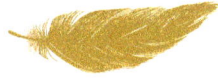

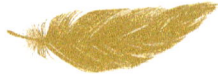

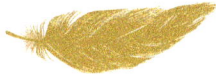

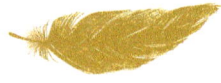

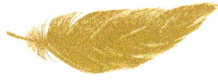

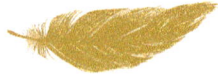

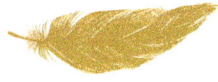

LivingUpp
A Lifestyle Design Company

300+ Self-Care Activities

Systemic: How you eat, move, rest and prevent illnesses

Rate your 8

Maintain a healthy weight

Limit sugar

Practice deep breathing

Wash your hands

Track your menstrual cycle and symptoms

Open a Health Savings Account (HSA)

Get a flu shot

Enjoy a fermented food

Take a walk in the woods

Go paddleboarding

Toss expired over-the-counter medications

Moisturize your skin

Follow safe food handling practices

Practice safe sex

Plan a picnic

Bake something

Run a marathon

Make a list of questions to ask your doctor

See a dermatologist

Try reflexology

Work with a registered dietitian

Try a new exercise

Revamp your skincare routine

Go for a swim

Buy a new pillow

Take a Pilates class

Hire a coach

Try a new recipe

Clean out your refrigerator

Change your air filter

Get acupuncture

Pack your lunch

Exfoliate your skin

Run a 5k

Use a sugar scrub

Have a healthy snack

Take a walk with a friend

Enjoy a mocktail

Go meatless

Get a stand-up desk

Complete a living will

Care for your feet

Get a scalp massage

Do strength training exercises

Take a cooking class

Plan a menu

Get a manicure

Get a fluoride treatment

Buy a water filter

Organize your recipes

Quit tobacco

Buy new gym clothes

Have a pharmacist review your medications

Take a self-defense class

Get vaccinated

Give blood

Go kayaking

Buy a new mattress

Use a pressure cooker

Prepare a 3-day emergency kit

Buy new tennis shoes

Drink enough water

Take medications as prescribed

Schedule a walking meeting

Get a pedicure

Visit a fruit stand

Apply sunscreen

Volunteer at a community garden

Ferment pickles

Hire a personal trainer

Go canoeing

Sleep in

Get a massage

Build a treadmill workstation

Enjoy a cup of tea

Unwind in a hot tub

Floss

Set a bedtime alarm

Shop the farmers' market

Meditate

Create a personal medical record

Eat more colors

Make a grocery shopping list

Get CPR certified

Take a hike

Get a mammogram

Sit in silence

Cry

Get a health screening

Get a facial

Eat something green

Go cycling

Drink enough water

Walk a dog

Take a nap

Schedule preventive exams

Say no

Use an iron skillet

Get an annual physical

Go for a run

Assemble a first-aid kit

Take a tai chi class

Make bone broth

Make a smoothie

Use a foam roller

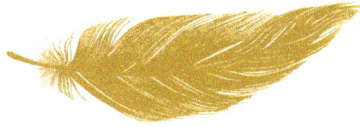

Systemic: How you eat, move, rest and prevent illnesses

Change your sheets

Eat 5 (to 9) servings of fruits and vegetables each day

Make homemade soup

Be the director of your healthcare

Eat breakfast

Shop around for health insurance plans

Ask for copies of your medical records

Take a soothing bath

Go to the gym

Go berry picking

Go to the dentist

Soak in Epsom salts

Take a yoga class

Take a dance class

Take a Barre class

Stretch

Get an eye exam

Emotive: How you express yourself and manage emotions

Rate your 8

Say thank you

Practice deep breathing

Talk about what you DO want rather than what you don't

Adopt a pet

Join Toastmasters

Learn the art of bonsai

Learn crochet or knitting

Make a scrapbook

Get a pedicure

Go to the symphony

Know your emotional triggers

Share your story

Establish a new morning ritual

Have your house professionally cleaned

Cuddle

Get a manicure

Enjoy a sunset

Get a scalp massage

Create a self-care survival plan

Listen to the ocean

Speak up

Take a warm shower

Listen to music

Join a support group

Get a massage

Write a letter of gratitude

Float a river

Relax at the spa

Write in a journal

Relax by a fire

Watch a funny movie

Work with a therapist

Enjoy a cup of tea

Write poetry

Unwind in a hot tub

Take an art class

Meditate

Journal affirmations

Relax with aromatherapy

Accept what is

Volunteer at the food bank

Snuggle with pets

Write a letter of gratitude

Be kind

Downsize your belongings

Go to the beach

Sit in silence

Cry

Make a list of things you love

Make a list of things you're grateful for

Turn off social media notifications

Celebrate your successes

Start a blog

Walk a dog

Take a nap

Prune your inner circle

Set healthy boundaries

Laugh

Say no

Learn to play a musical instrument

Ask for help

Give a gift

Take something off your to-do list

Perform a random act of kindness

Create a vision board

Go for a run

Take a tai chi class

Attend a live music event

Take the day off

Take a soothing bath

Apologize

Color

Sing

Take a yoga class

Take a dance class

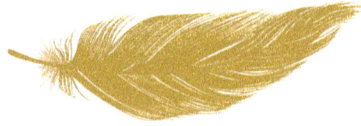

Luminescent: How you illuminate your inner truth

Rate your 8

Identify your core values

Get a haircut

Ask for what you need

Identify how you want to feel

Work with a therapist

Take an art class

Work with a wardrobe stylist

Vote

Understand your personality

Know your strengths

Read old journals

Meditate

Journal affirmations

Hire a coach

Accept what is

Share your story

Do your best

Create a capsule wardrobe

Be kind

Change your mind

Speak up

Read scripture

Make a scrapbook

Sit in silence

Get clear about what you want to do, have, be, and feel

Make a list of things you love

Start a blog

Write a book

Set healthy boundaries

Say no

Get your makeup done professionally

Create a vision board

Take a tai chi class

Establish a personal brand

Check with your health plan to see what's covered

Take a yoga class

Take a dance class

Financial: How you allocate your resources

Rate your 8

Define what your "enough" looks like

Become debt-free

Ask for what you need

Downsize your belongings

Work with a financial adviser

Check with your health plan to see what's covered

Create a capsule wardrobe

Get clear about what you want to do, have, be, and feel

Have leftovers for dinner

Say no

Cook at home

Reduce spending

Fund a retirement account

Open a Health Savings Account (HSA)

Cancel a membership

Create a budget

Own less stuff

Use a money management app

Hire a CPA

Create a vision board

Get a new certification

Create a last will & testament

Pay bills online

Go window shopping

Schedule a regular review of your finances

Ask for generic medications when possible

Shop around for insurance plans

Review your medical statements

Cognitive: How you think, learn and manage your mindset

Rate your 8

Set healthy goals

Expect good things

Release expectations

Drink alcohol in moderation if at all

Weigh the pros and cons

before making a decision

Establish a new morning ritual

Research

Overcome a fear

Learn to sail

Write in a journal

Listen to a podcast

Create a self-care survival plan

Learn crochet or knitting

Think about what you DO want rather than what you don't

Work with a therapist

Get clear about what you want to do, have, be, and feel

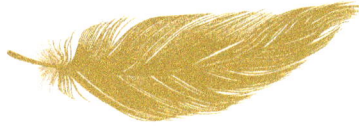

Cognitive: How you think, learn and manage your mindset

Work a puzzle

Go to a bookstore

Write poetry

Hire a coach

Create a bucket list

Learn to play a musical instrument

Join a book club

Visit the library

Meditate

Think the best of everyone

Take a continuing education class

Journal affirmations

Explore new possibilities

Accept what is

Be kind

Plan your week ahead of time

Define what your "enough" looks like

Change your mind

Sit in silence

Make a list of things you love

Turn off social media notifications

Schedule a planning retreat

Drink enough water

Start a blog

Get a new certification

Attend a workshop

Walk a dog

Read old journals

Take a nap

Write a book

Set healthy boundaries

Say no

Ask for help

Listen to an audio book

Set weekly goals

Vote

Read a book

Create a vision board

Be the director of your healthcare

Eat breakfast

Take the day off

Create a manifestation space

Establish a personal brand

Take a yoga class

Travel to another country

Update your insurance policy beneficiaries

Aptitudinal: How you contribute to the world

Rate your 8

Take an art class

Delegate a task

Work with a business coach

Take a continuing education class

Ask for what you need

Take something off your to-do list

Work with a career coach

Make a list of essential tasks

Create a manifestation space

Join Toastmasters

Do your best

Share your story

Plan your week ahead of time

Use a planner

Learn to play a musical instrument

Hire a coach

Make a list of things you love

Designate times to check email

Listen actively

Schedule a planning retreat

Establish a new morning ritual

Start a blog

Attend a workshop

Speak up

Write a book

Say no

Find a mentor

Set weekly goals

Create a vision board

Take the day off

Get a new certification

Start a bullet journal

Establish a personal brand

Track your goals

Build something

Download a health-related app

Take an online course

Make a list of your top 5 goals each week

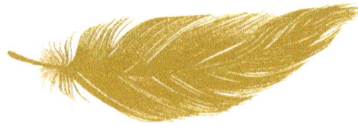

Relational: How you connect with others

Rate your 8

Say thank you

Develop a family emergency plan

Understand your personality

Practice deep breathing

Cuddle

Be an organ donor

Practice safe sex

Help a neighbor with a project

Ask for what you need

Meet new people

Forgive

Work with a therapist

Share your story

Get family photos updated

Spend time with friends

Hold space for someone

Join a book club

Plan a picnic

Think the best of everyone

Take a walk with a friend

Know your emotional triggers

Volunteer at the food bank

Get CPR certified

Write a letter of gratitude

Speak up

Reconnect with an old friend

Plan a date night

Organize a gathering

Give blood

Be kind

Ask for forgiveness

Turn off social media notifications

Listen actively

Join a support group

Start a blog

Prune your inner circle

Grow your community

Set healthy boundaries

Say no

Buy coffee for a stranger

Ask for help

Complete a living will

Give a gift

Perform a random act of kindness

Be the director of your healthcare

Join a civic organization

Create a last will & testament

Have coffee with a friend

Ask questions

Schedule a walking meeting

Find a mentor

Join Toastmasters

Apologize

Spend quality time with family

Establish a personal brand

Travel to another country

Volunteer at a community garden

Update your insurance policy beneficiaries

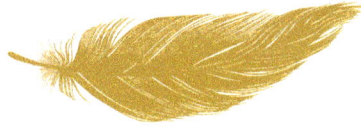

Environmental: How you harmonize with nature, your community and your personal spaces

Rate your 8

Donate something you no longer need

Tidy up your workspace

Take a walk in the woods

Adopt a pet

Have your house professionally cleaned

Plan a trip

Go paddleboarding

Work with a permaculture designer

Enjoy a sunset

Listen to the ocean

Go fishing

Use reusable grocery bags

Repurpose something

Fold laundry

Take a road trip

Go on an adventure

Learn to sail

Play in the snow

Relax with aromatherapy

Recycle

Volunteer at the food bank

Snuggle with pets

Use a composter

Get CPR certified

Spend time in the Garden

Take a hike

Smell the roses

Go to the symphony

Visit a museum

Downsize your belongings

Go to the beach

Sit in silence

Walk a dog

Buy a houseplant

Change your sheets

Take a self-defense class

Plant a tree

Attend a live music event

Go sightseeing

Go berry picking

Take a shorter shower

Use a water filter

Travel to another country

Clean your yoga mat

Volunteer at a community garden

Join a civic organization

Go camping

Go canoeing

Buy a new pillow

Go for a swim

Go stargazing

Float a river

Learn the art of bonsai

Clean out your refrigerator

Change your air filter

Organize a closet

Create a music playlist

Make a donation to a charity

Put together an emergency kit for your car

Create a manifestation space

Vote

Rearrange furniture

Make your bed

Bonus

Do you want more ease and better health?

Head on over to LivingUpp.com/Bonus
to receive your free gifts!

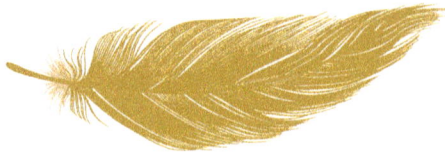

www.ingramcontent.com/pod-product-compliance
Lightning Source LLC
Chambersburg PA
CBHW040832040426
42336CB00034B/3421